MW01436835

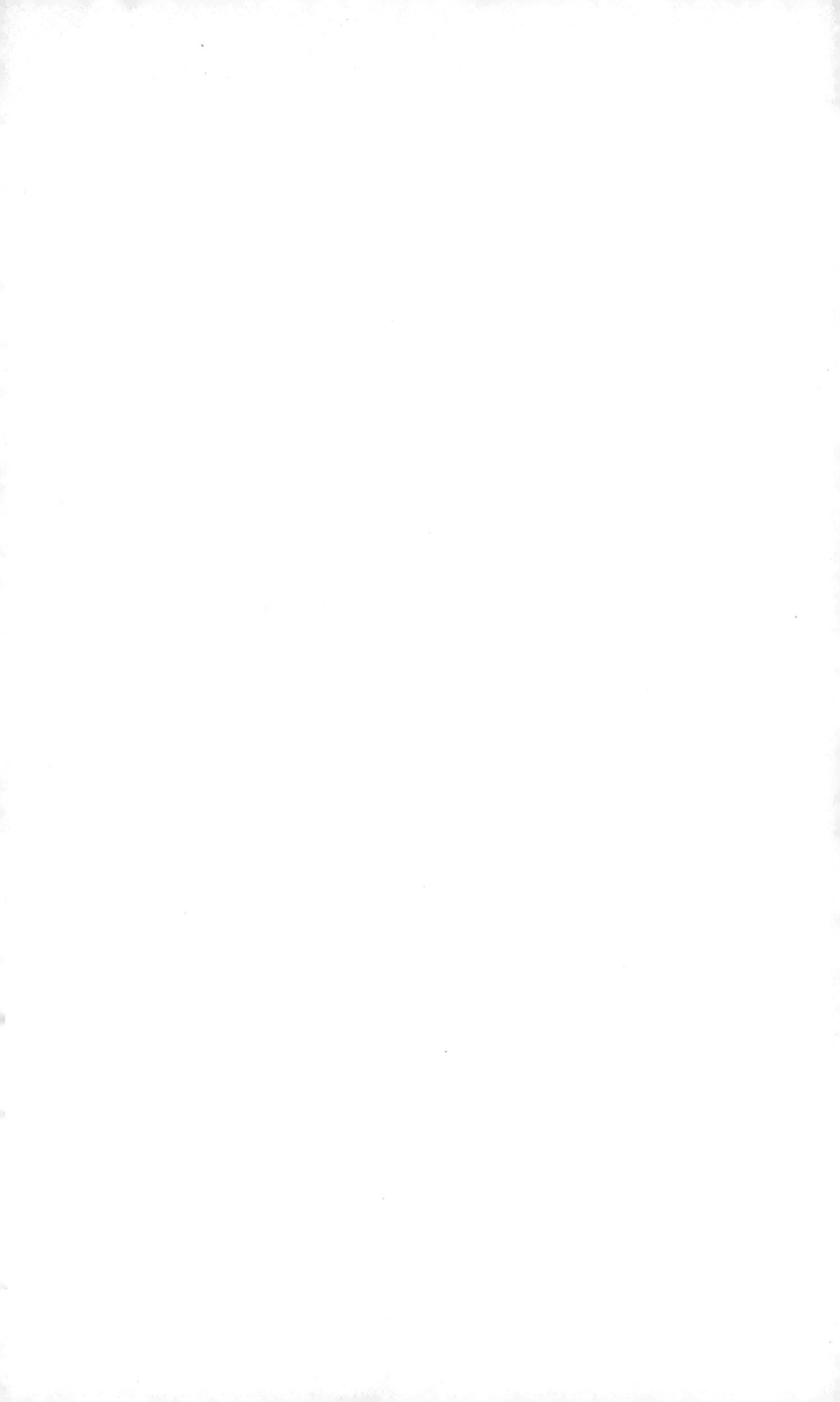

SCARED OF THAT

Living While Dying of AIDS

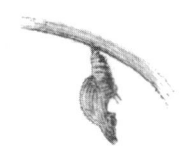

Sylvia Zingeser

Ariela Press
Portland, Oregon

Some poems have appeared in *Alchemy*, Portland Community College Literary Magazine, Portland, Oregon: "Fearful Hierarchies" and "Throwing Out Tea Bags." Others have appeared in *Mercury*, a quarterly arts and literature supplement to *The Bridge*, Portland Community College newspaper, Portland, Oregon: "Spider Babies," "Three AIDS Poems," "Breathing: An Unrealized Meditation," "Driving Home," and "I Sat On Tears."

Copyright © by Sylvia Zingeser

All rights reserved. Printed in the United States of America. No part of this book may be used or reproduced in any manner whatsoever without written permission except for brief reviews or articles relevant to subject matter. All inquiries should be addressed to Ariela Press, P. O. Box 82832, Portland, Oregon 97219-0832.

First Edition, 1997

Library of Congress Catalog Number: 97-94213
ISBN: 0-9659451-0-3

Sylvia Zingeser, poems and short stories
Linda Thomson, cover and book design
Sandra Kovtun, *POLYPHARMACOPEIA* collage
Sandra Anton Gee, documentary photographs, 1988-1997
Jon Leon, illustrations
Judy Horowitz, calligraphy
Tsispora Diment, Hebrew translation
Mark Dewey, Barbara Thyne, Stephen Weed, Adam Wunn, Diana Yates, PrintPaks, and *The Woman's Journal*, computer assistance

Collage made from Aaron Walters' medication bottles he'd saved for the last two years of his life.

Printed by Pioneer Printing, Inc., Newport, Oregon in association with Oregon Coast Rural Information Service Cooperative (OCRISC), Waldport, Oregon.

Introduction

When I first started to write about the AIDS journey of my eldest son, Aaron Walters, I did not know where it would lead me. Now I realize it is more than an account of someone who was born gay and died from AIDS.
We live in an era when medicine is expected to heal all diseases, ailments, and injuries. Western medicine has extended the lives of people who have developed terminal illnesses. All too often, the physically well pull away from those who are sick or dying. The notion of dying as a part of living is not well accepted.
People who pull back from a dying loved one deny themselves the opportunity to work through their loss. Through my own grieving, I came to understand that I can share with others the importance of being present in some way with loved ones who are debilitated or who are dying.
Scared of That shows what it takes to stay alive. The cover photo of the collage depicts the medicine required to keep going for two years. Taking this much medicine is not unique to AIDS. Many other illnesses require exorbitant amounts of medicine as well.
Aaron wanted to share his experience so that people who are sexually active would have a candid look at what it's like to live an AIDS life. With education, AIDS can be avoided. When his health allowed, he spoke for AIDS agencies on safe sex and funding for people with AIDS (PWA's). He didn't know such a disease existed when he was first infected, which occurred probably in 1978 or 1979.
Grieving takes time. It's an illness all its own. One doesn't have to forget; one never does. But a person can move on to enjoy life again. That was Aaron's wish for me.
I pass on his wish in *Scared of That*.

DELIVERY AND TAKE-OUT MENU

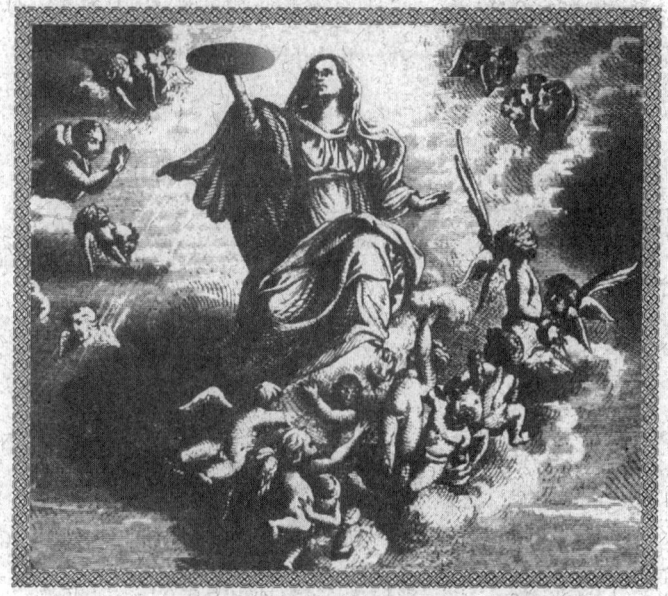

"ANOTHER PERFECT PIZZA!"

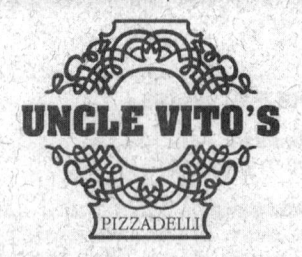

UNCLE VITO'S
PIZZADELLI

at bush & powell streets in san francisco

Thank You Sandy and Merle Kovtun for the many wonderful, healthy meals you sent to me while I was taking care of Aaron.

Acknowledgments

Many thanks to my instructors—Michael McDowell, Reva Leeman, Linda Warwick, and Bill Siverly of Portland Community College, Sylvania Campus, Portland, Oregon—who have encouraged me to write. A special thanks to Michael McDowell for patiently editing my work and taking a great amount of time to do so.

My gratitude and thanks to Rabbi Eric Weiss for his spiritual guidance and help that I cannot put into words.

Many thanks to Sandy Kovtun, Aaron's practical support volunteer from Jewish Family *and* Children's Services (JFCS) in San Francisco, who was truly there for us both emotionally and practically.

Thank you to Jody Reiss, JFCS Aids Project Coordinator, for her devotion and expertise. To Rachel Kasselman, JFCS AIDS Volunteer Coordinator, for connecting Aaron with The Chicken Soupers, a volunteer group that provides homemade kosher meals to PWA's, and for making the perfect match between practical support person and client.

A special thank you to Ann Green, the one family member who understood Aaron's pain and gave him spiritual nourishment and hope from the time of his AIDS diagnosis.

An enormous thank you to Sandra Anton Gee, who with great care documented with her photography as much of Aaron's life as possible while he was living in San Francisco. To Irving Hulteen, whom Aaron and I met at Coming Home Hospice, for critiquing and sharing insights.

A special thank you to Stephen Weed for the many hours he spent with electronic page layout. To Sara Wrench for critiquing and editing. To Orpha Barry, Carla Perry, Annalise Santiago, Linda Thomson, Barb Thyne, Dick Thyne, and Diana Yates for final preparation of the document for the printer.

Thank you to Grey Wolfe for her guidance and critiques.

Many thanks to Jon Leon for the illustrations of Aaron and the butterfly series. To Judy Horowitz for the Hebrew calligraphy and Tsispora Diment for the Hebrew translation of Ahavai Shalom.

Thank you to PrintPaks and *The Woman's Journal* for the use of their computer equipment.

Also, thank you to Alan Park for editing and Adam Wunn for computer assistance at the beginning of the project.

And thank you to Aaron's many wonderful friends, my friends, and our family, for their love and support.

Contents

Introduction   iii
Acknowledgments   v

I. San Francisco: 1990

Lookin' Too Good, An AIDS Poem	3
My Breakfast	4
Designer Dinner	7
Rose Water Bath	13
Chips, Flecks, and Fine Dust	16
Spider Babies	18
Limos	22
Exit Door	24
The Tan Plastic Bottle	25

II. Going Down: Spring, 1992

Three AIDS Poems	28
Queer as a Three Dollar Ruble	30
Trekking with Auntie Ann	31
Cody Comes to Dish	32
Kitchen Walls Talk	35
Russian/Ukrainian Steps	37
An Unlikely Dessert	38
Snap Trap	44
Breathing: An Unrealized Meditation	45
Waking Up to Die	47
Rainbow Butterfly	48
Metamorphosis	51

III. Universal Traveler: October 10, 1992

Fearful Hierarchies	58
No Clue	59
A Different Kind of Veteran	61
Driving Home	63
Love of Peace	65
A Gala Event for Sandy Kovtun	67
I Sat on Tears	69
Marlboro Spurs	70
Large Pink Duofold	71
April 9, 1996	72
Edward Scissorhands Bouquet	73
Throwing Out Tea Bags	74
Molecular Journeys	77
Glossary	78

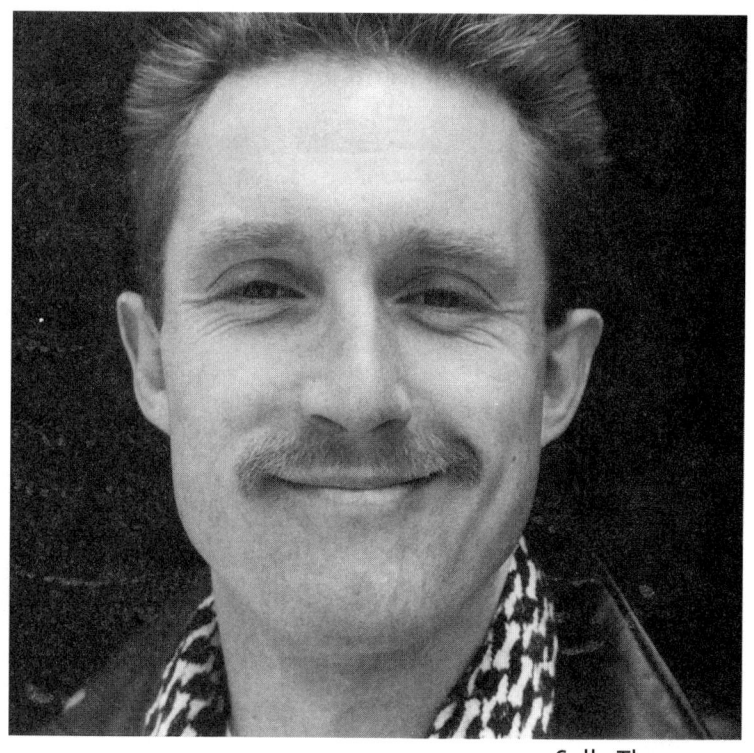

Sally Thompson

Aaron, who gave me many gifts—his friends, connections, and the courage to continue living.

Mom, just because I die doesn't mean you have to.

My eldest son was born gay . . .

I

San Francisco
Spring 1990

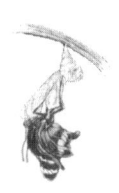

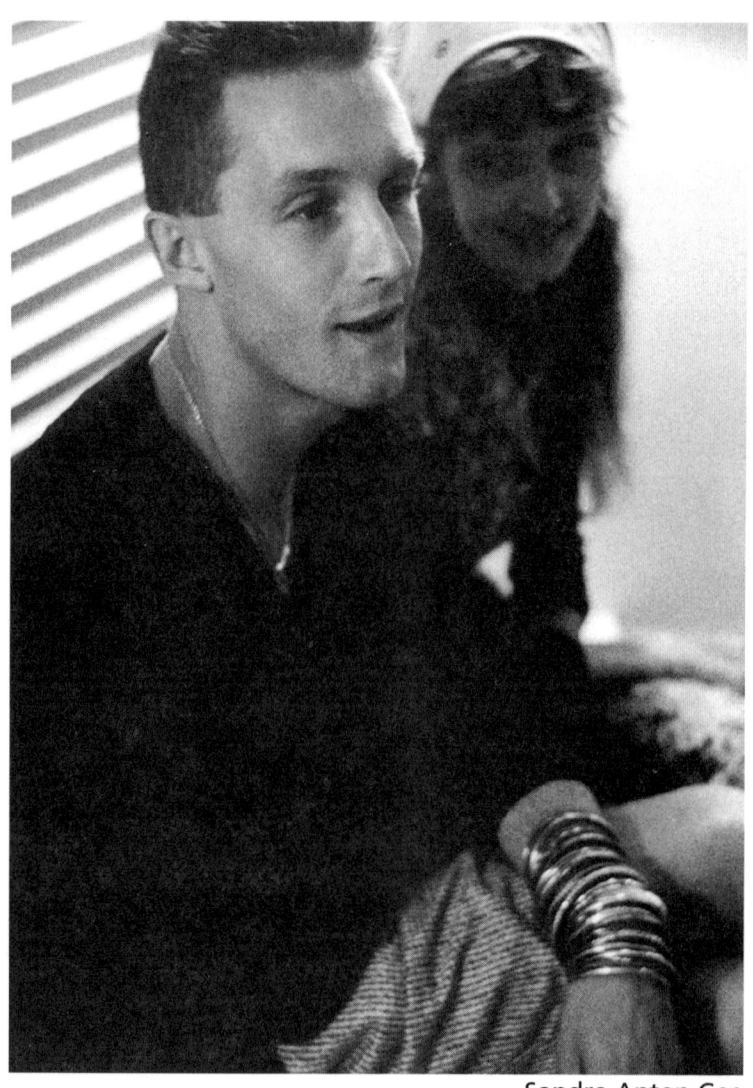

Sandra Anton Gee

Lookin' Too Good
An AIDS Poem

He looks healthy.
Don't you think
he should work?

He just wants someone
to take care of him.
I know that's it.

She looks in perfect health.
Why not work?
What's her problem anyway?

Lazy, I'm sure.
I know that's it.
Don't you agree?

She looks good.
He looks good.
They're lookin' so good.

My Breakfast

I feel the warm gentle rays of the sun engulf my body as I begin to stir about on the futon. The courtyard of my red brick apartment building is now filled with fresh morning light and the flapping of doves' wings signals another day launched.
I'm thankful for the sun, for it's much better to wake up to than Minnesota snow or Oregon rain. Times like this make me realize the decision to move to San Francisco was a good one.
Weariness and fatigue, my constant companions, make it hard for me to get up. I look at the clock. Six a.m., and I calculate whether it's time to start breakfast. I rise gradually, hoping to prevent the dizziness that might otherwise occur. I reach for the slippers and put them on, then slowly begin to push myself up from the futon. I feel like a little old man as I try to stand upright. All I can negotiate is a bent stature. I shuffle to the bathroom. "This is not normal for a thirty-year-old male," I say to myself.
With one thought in mind, I move toward the kitchen for my self-prescribed medication, a first morning cigarette. To me, this keeps my priorities straight. It's one addiction I haven't conquered, much to my doctors' regrets.
Cigarettes are best when accompanied with a good cup of coffee, so I'll make myself a small pot of French roast. It's truly a comfort to alternate a swig of coffee with a drag from my Winston while I sit by my kitchen window and watch the doves take wing from their favorite tree, a tall pine that nearly fills the courtyard below.

Today I have two pieces of toast, unlike most days, before I prepare the breakfast that really counts. As the last corner of the toast fills my mouth, I mentally prepare myself for the main course.

With considerable effort, I slide my feet to the cupboard and pull out the black bowl. From the center shelf, I remove a cylindrical brown plastic bottle filled with white elliptical pills that have blue bands around their middles. Three AZT's, one hundred milligram capsules, are needed for the morning appetizer. The Acyclovir is an all-sea-blue capsule, two hundred milligrams. I place two of these in the black bowl with the AZT's—both are antiviral drugs. Next is the Fluconazole, a one hundred milligram bright pink, triangular-shaped tablet. This is an antifungal agent. Bactrim DS, the one I dread the most, causes a nausea that builds up in my stomach like the churning of a great typhoon at sea. It is an oversized chalk-white tablet that contains eight hundred milligrams of Sulfa, plus one hundred sixty milligrams of Trimethoprim, given for the bronchitis and pneumonia I continually fight. The tablet is so large that most of the time it sticks to the back of my throat when I try to swallow it. One Empirin number four, a potent analgesic, seems to work the best on the kind of pain I have in the joints and skin of my feet and legs. Then comes two tiny half hot pink and half white twenty-five milligram Benadryl capsules. These are for the incredible itching which is due, I'm convinced, to all the other drugs that I'm putting into my body. And how could I forget, as if all this isn't enough, the new one that was just added to my breakfast, Atarax, a tiny black dot of a pill in generic form, twenty-five milligrams. It helps relieve the itching and the horrible nausea that looms over me every morning.

Now my breakfast is finally ready. The pills arrange themselves in kaleidoscope with each movement of the black bowl. I shuffle to the table and begin to devour them, these life extending entities, as though they were a bowl of oatmeal. I would prefer the oatmeal.

The pills are consumed and I top my breakfast off with another cigarette and a cup of coffee while I gaze into the courtyard below. A new day has been initiated once again.

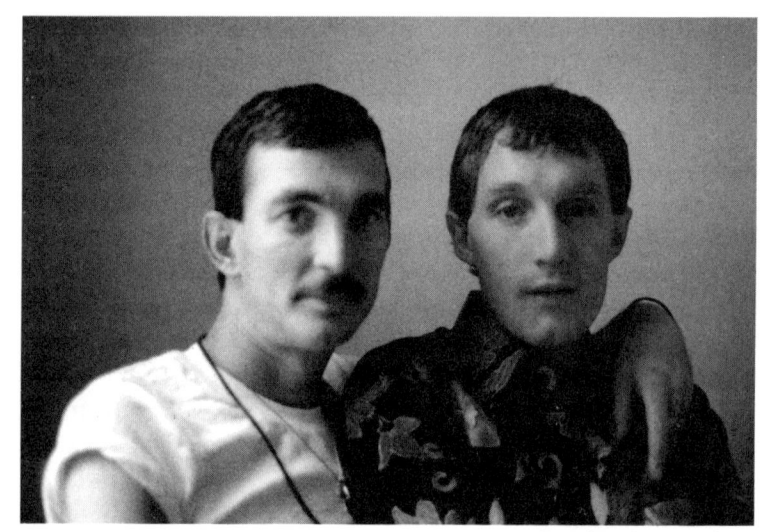

Sandra Anton Gee

Designer Dinner

My mom arrived at the front door of my apartment building in high style. I had put her onto the airport limousine service; it's cheaper and I wouldn't worry as much about her. She's not a big city girl. Until she arrived, it was hard for me to visualize her bumming around the streets of San Francisco with me and Bob, but that's what she did. I buzzed her in the main door of the apartment building from my phone. It was good to see her and she was cool about Bob. I knew she would be. Bob has AIDS. So do I. And we're going to catch an early dinner this evening.

I met Bob on Gay Pride Day in the Castro in San Francisco. That was a month ago. He was sick and I could tell he was close to checkout time.

I was standing in an incredibly long line to use the bathroom in the Castro Station bar, one of the local leather bars on Castro Street, when this tall brown-eyed beauty came in and tried to go ahead of everyone. As he pushed ahead, people started to yell at him, "Go to the back of the line." He begged to go ahead, but no one listened.

"Get a life, girlfriends. Can't you see he's having a problem?" I said as I stepped out of line. "Do you need some help?"

"Yeah," he said.

"My name is Aaron. What's your name?" I slipped my arm around him.

"I'm Bob," he said. "Boy, I'm glad you're here."

"Looks like you've got a little problem."

"Yeah," he said. His face turned pink as I grabbed his arm. We muscled our way into a stall and I started to help him get cleaned up as much as possible.

"Maybe you should go home and get some clean clothes?"

"Would you go with me?"

"Where's your home?"

"Sausalito."

"Way out there?" I said. Bob looked down with his brown

eyes fixed on me. "Do you have a car?"

"No," he said.

"You don't take the bus, do you?"

"Yeah."

"That's a long trip." Bob gave me a look I couldn't say no to. "Oh, all right, where do we catch the bus?"

We pushed through the crowds and waited for the number twenty-four Divisadero bus that would connect us with the Golden Gate Transit on Lombard Street. I was pretty pumped up before the parade but my energy level had started to drop off. Still, there was something about Bob that made me want to go with him. I recognized the feeling right away. It was strong, like the pull of the ocean floor that creeps up a sandy beach and latches onto someone's ankles, carrying them back to its heart, claiming them for itself. I've waited a long time for that special someone but nothing's stuck yet. Now I have AIDS stuff going on inside me. Who would want to get hooked up with someone who has AIDS?

It was late afternoon by now and the trip across the Golden Gate Bridge has a certain air of peacefulness, a sense of connection with worlds unknown to me. Bob reached over to pick up my hand and I quickly slipped my hand into his, squeezing it gently. We'd do this together, I thought, the AIDS thing.

"Do you live by yourself?" I asked.

"No, I live with my ex-lover, Mark. In the garage."

"That sounds awful."

"It's O.K. He has a new lover. You'll meet him. His name is Francisco. It's a nickname."

"With a name like that, he has to be interesting," I said. "Does Mark have AIDS?"

"No, he's not sick. He says he's going to get tested one of these days."

"He'd better get tested soon, because if he's positive, he needs to line up a good doctor and make some decisions about his treatment," I said. "What about Mark's new lover, has he been tested?"

"I don't know." Bob said.

"Uhmm."

The bus made its way onto the freeway that follows the

northern shoreline of the bay. We hardly noticed the curves that swayed us back and forth into each other.

"God, what a mess," I said. "This place has real potential to be something. What happened?"

"Oh, Mark's going to landscape it," Bob said. "He's a landscape architect, but he's so busy that there isn't enough time to do his own yard."

"I see," I said while I scrutinized the surroundings closer. Bob led the way through the unkempt yard to the dark garage where he lived. Clothes were thrown about, the bed was unmade with covers piled high in places. Dirty cups and glasses sat intermingled with brown plastic medication bottles on makeshift end tables. "I'd better go home before it gets any later," I said.

Bob looked wistfully in my direction and asked, "Aaron, can I come home with you?"

I was a little nervous when I called my mom the next time.

"Mom, I have something to tell you," I said. "I don't know how to explain this, but I met this really cute guy at the Gay Pride Parade last weekend. His name is Bob."

"I'm listening," she said.

"He came home with me," I said. "He doesn't want to go back to his place. He's not happy there and he's sick. I don't think he's going to live much longer. It's really sad."

"Where's his family? Are they involved with his care?"

"I talked with his ex-lover and he said that the family kind of kissed him off," I said. "Apparently, the mother caused all kinds of problems between him and Bob. His mother lives in Florida."

"Oh, great," she said. "The most understanding state in the Union."

"Yeah. Pretty bad, huh?" I said. "Is it O.K. with you if Bob stays with me? I know you're paying the rent. I feel guilty putting you in this position, but...."

"I'm just concerned that you'll get sick," she said. "You know what's coming down the pike."

"Yeah," I said. "But it's too late. He has one of the worst

9

cases of dementia I've seen yet. He's been here three days and it's a lot worse than I realized. He's actually picked me to live with."

"Does your social worker know what's happening? What did your doctor say?"

"They know," I said. "They have some of the same concerns you have, but they know that once I make up my mind, that's how it is. Mom, when are you coming down? I could use your help. Do you mind?"

"I was planning on the third week of July. How does that sound?"

The weather was perfect—not too hot, not too cool. I made Bob get dressed every day and go for walks in the neighborhood. He had graduated to a cane and I had to watch him as if he were a small child. Sometimes he tried to shake me and go off on his own. He constantly wanted to smoke but I limited his cigarettes because his lungs were full of infection. He would smoke nonstop if I let him. And I had to keep medications locked up because he just took pills to take them. He no longer understood exactly why he took the pills. He was a handful.

"Isn't he sweet, Mom?" I asked. "I think he's really cute, but he drives me nuts at the same time."

"I can see that you do care for him," she said. "He gives you a reason to keep going, don't you think?"

"You're probably right."

Bob got excited when we got him ready to go out to my favorite Japanese restaurant. He hassled me for a cigarette as we walked down Geary. He knew it was not time for another one, but he tried anyway. I told him no and he pouted for about three blocks, lagging way behind and sliding his feet as we slowly walked on.

"Aaron, won't you give me a cigarette?" Bob asked, his lower lip protruding. He looked down at the sidewalk covered with bits of paper and garbage. He saw a cigarette butt and reached to pick it up and place it in his mouth.

"Bob, that's really dirty," my mom said. "You could get sick if you put that in your mouth."

"No, I won't." He brushed it off. "See, it's clean now. Aaron, give me a light. What do you say? O.K.?"

"How about if I make you a deal?" she said. "After dinner you can have a cigarette. What do you say? O.K.?"

Bob eyed the dirty cigarette butt and then looked back at my mom.

"Promise?" Bob asked.

"Promise."

"O.K.," Bob said. And we started to walk again. Bob seemed satisfied with the agreement. A couple more blocks and we were there.

The restaurant was big enough to hold about twenty people. The tables lined one wall and the cooks and sushi bar were on the opposite side. The ceiling was dropped so that tall people had to stoop to walk. Bob is tall so he had to stoop. Everybody who worked there was Japanese. I was a regular and they knew I wanted tempura. They brought us miso and we picked out the tiny chunks of tofu with our chopsticks and drank the rest. Dinner arrived on rectangular plastic trays that imitated inlaid wood. The vegetables and shrimp took on new shapes that looked like golden laced animals bedded down in slivers of cabbage and carrots. And before we had got started with our designer dinner, Bob had struck up a conversation with the couple at the next table.

"Hi," Bob said to the couple. They were smoking. "Can I have a cigarette?"

Before my mom and I could stop Bob, the woman handed him a cigarette. He jumped up from the table and scurried as fast as he could into the bathroom and locked the door. I followed close behind.

"Bob, unlock the door," I said.

"Just a minute," Bob said. "I'll be out in a minute."

I began to get irritated. I could hear him start to cough and the smell of cigarette smoke eased its way out from underneath the door.

"Bob, put that cigarette out," I said. "You're going to start coughing. Do you hear me?"

"Yeah, yeah," he said.

"Come out right now. I'm getting really angry with you."

Bob opened the door and glared at me. "You're really misbehaving," I said. I followed him back to the table. Bob sulked. The couple at the next table stared at us.

"Aaron's mad at me," Bob said to my mom. "He won't let me have a cigarette."

"How about a cigarette when we get home where you can sit and enjoy it?" my mom asked.

"Promise?"

"Promise."

"O.K."

Rose Water Bath

When Bob started to cough one night, I knew I'd have to take him into the emergency room at Mt. Zion Hospital and fight with him and the medical staff. Bob didn't think there was anything wrong with him; he just wanted to have another cigarette. I told the doctor we couldn't get the cough under control and I was afraid he had pneumocystis. They put him in an examining room and did the usual things: took his temperature and blood pressure, drew his blood, and asked him how he felt.

"Fine," he said. He didn't look fine to me and he didn't act fine either. Besides, he was running a temperature.

"Well, Bob, you're better," the doctor said. "Your white cell count was a thousand a few days ago, but now it's two thousand."

"I think he's got an infection," I said. But what do I know? I haven't been to medical school. Bob said he was O.K. and that he felt fine even though he couldn't breathe well and he choked up when he tried to sleep. They sent him home anyway. That was on a Sunday afternoon. The next day they hospitalized him; he had some kind of an infection, just like I thought.

After Bob got out of the hospital, he and I shuffled to doctor's appointments and made mini excursions up Polk Street for cups of coffee, cigarettes, and small bouquets of roses. I had to keep a close eye on him or he'd slip away from me.

It was after the first of August and Bob was loaded with five twenty dollar bills. I left him home alone while I went to the AIDS clinic. He was getting too weak to make unnecessary treks.

Bob decided he needed a little drink so he grabbed his cane and went out. He wasn't more than a half a block away from our apartment when some homeless looking guy pushed him into a building wall and pulled a knife on him.

"Gimme your cash. Now!" the guy said.

"All right, all right. Just a minute." Bob pulled his wallet out and the guy grabbed it, took the money out, and threw the wallet on the sidewalk before running. Bob leaned on his cane as he reached for his wallet.

One night I woke up and Bob wasn't there. I sat up and called out for Bob. There was no answer. I pushed off the futon. I could see light flickering from the kitchen. I poked my head in.

"Bob, what are you doing!" I shouted. "Are you trying to burn the house down?" Forty candles, nearly a whole box, stood erect in their own wax on the kitchen window sill; the flames waved at us. "Those are my Shabbas candles, Bob. You can't just light them."

"Look, Aaron, aren't they pretty?" Bob said as he smiled real big.

Bob's cough got worse. Blood red spots started to pop up on his legs and arms and it looked to me like he was starting to go down for sure. His sister, Sandy, and her lover, Lynn, came to hang out with us.

When his mother came to stay, I saw the way she looked as she laid her eyes on him. Her eyes widened and the cheeks sank in around the mouth. I watched as she held her breath. Only a mother could have a look like that.

His mother started crocheting an afghan for him. It was red, gray, white, and black and she finished it in five days. We put the afghan over him.

"Ooooh, I like that," he said. "Aaron, can I have a cigarette?" Every time a cigarette slipped out of Bob's fingers, it dropped onto the afghan to burn holes in it.

Now that Bob was with me, his sisters and brother, aunts and uncles, started to call and send things we needed to take care of him: sheets, towels, blankets, things we were short on. Every day we would get phone calls and cards.

Bob could hardly push off of our queen-sized futon so we moved it into the large walk-in closet and brought in a big hospital bed. He got weaker and the pain increased in his legs and feet. His lungs continued to fill with infection and fluid. The pain increased in his joints and chest so the doctor started him on morphine. Now he was an official hospice client of the Visiting Nurse's Hospice of San Francisco (VNH).

Bob's mother went back knowing it was the last time she'd ever see him. I felt bad for her. I thought about how my own mother would feel when it was my turn.

Bob was the love of my life. He was the one I was waiting for and I only got to be with him for two months, but it felt like we had been together forever.

I sat up night and day with Bob for the next three weeks before he died. We cooed to one another as I cleaned him up, tried to feed him, and give him medicine to kill the infection. I finally gave in to his smoking. I'd light a cigarette for him and one for me. He became so weak that he could hardly get a good drag, but we'd blow smoke at each other anyway and then giggle.

The day that Bob died, VNH sent an attendant named David Cardenas. He wore a black T-shirt and a silver chain with a carved crystal that hung down like a big tear drop. He had a bottle of rose water in his hand.

Bill, Bob's Shanti Project buddy, made coffee for us and sat in the kitchen while I held Bob in my arms. Even though Bob was six feet tall, I felt like I was holding a small child. I looked at his face as he took the last breath. I wept. It was early afternoon.

"Would you like to clean Bob up now?" David asked as he put his hand on my shoulder.

"Yeah," I said.

An hour had already passed by. David took the bottle of rose water and poured it in a monkey pod dish. He handed me a clean cloth; we dipped them into the rose water and began to wash Bob's malleable flesh. Bill put a stick of sandalwood incense in a wooden holder and lit it. The smoke curled around Bob's head and encircled us.

Chips, Flecks, and Fine Dust

August 1990:
Pink turns to tan. Red blood cells turn rust-brown.
Ferric—Bob back to his salt of the earth origins.
Hematite—five-six on the Mohs scale.
Chip of black: Is it silicone?
Chips of bone: Knitted calcite hexagons.
The crematorium has mortared and pestled
Bob to flecks and fine dust.

December 1990:
In my backpack, Bob sifts
in a gold foil cardboard box,
stuffed under the seat in front of me,
where I can keep an eye on him

Delta all the way:
San Francisco to San Diego,
to pick up Sandy, Bob's sister,
and her lover, Lynn,
and on to Miami.

Christmas in the sun:
We deep sea fish for some fun.
And next day Bob's family meet at Blowing Rock
to scatter him off a spit
at the Sailor's House of Refuge,
Indian River Inlet, Florida.

Wearing Bob:
We open the gold foil cardboard box, scooped
handfuls of chips, flecks, and fine dust
and gently threw them toward the Atlantic.
The wind caught Bob and pitched him
back into our hair and faces.
Daisies and bougainvillea floated where we threw them.
They swayed like rocking dinghies,
and the chips, flecks, and fine dust mixed with the water.

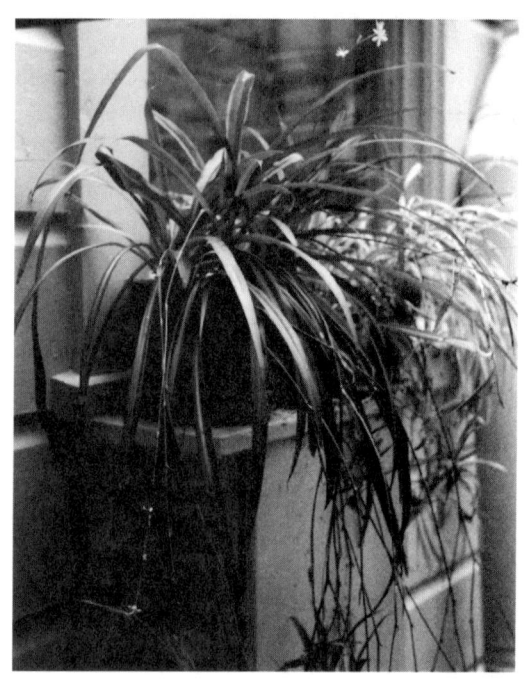

Sandra Anton Gee

Spider Babies

A green gallon
plastic planter
filled
with spider plants
sits
on a window sill
of a second floor
apartment,
number 207,
Rex Arms,
at the corner
of Polk
and Geary,
San Francisco.
Strong projections,

one-third
the size
of an ordinary
pencil,
protrude up
through
a mesh
of lush greenery.
White flowers
like tiny stars
in a galaxy
form clusters
and dangle
from the long
protrusions
as they drop
out the window,
hang suspended,
and nearly touch
the courtyard below.
Colors of green
vary as sunlight
filters
through two
tall trees,
one a fir,
the other
a sparse pine.
The aged red
brick wall
enlivens
the profuse
green
spider babies
tended
by the careful hands
of Aaron.
The aroma
of sandalwood incense

mixed
with Ultra Lite
Winston
cigarettes
floats
through the narrow
long
pointed
leaves
and out
the open window.

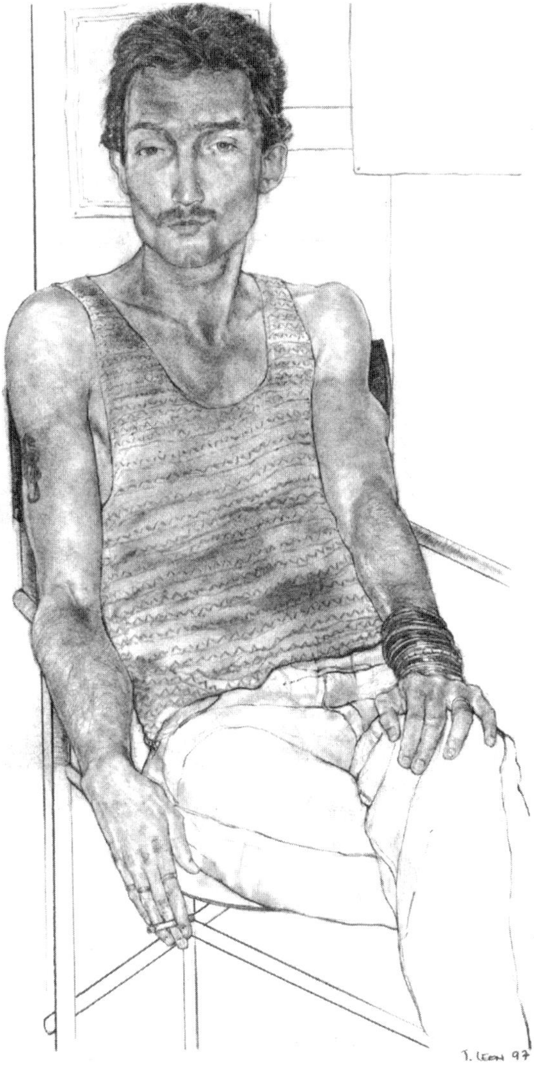
T. LEON 97

Limos

I watch bright lights
congested streets
rush,
rush by.

Limos
filled with businessmen
businesswomen
wives
husbands
world travelers
honeymooners
vacationers
mothers;
seldom fathers
to see their sons or daughters.

Limos
drop off clients.
First a luxurious hotel,
then a quaint one.
China Town, too.
I'm dropped off last
at the Rex Arms apartments
corner of Polk and Geary.
All around Reagan's homeless
and mentally ill stand.

Limos
drive me through this foreign place.
I watch my step,
won't look in people's eyes.
I push the buzzer
and think, hurry, let me in.
My son, so thin,
greets me with a smile and a kiss.
"It's O.K., Mom."
I say to him, "It's not O.K."

The driver looks at us.
We wave him on.
He'll be back in a few days
to pick me up
to take me away.

Exit Door

I quit counting the times I pass through the exit door
that faces east of a clinic's nurses' station
at Mt. Zion Hospital.

Each time I cross its threshold on my way
to the AIDS clinic, anxiety fills my chest travels
to my throat across my shoulders and down
into my arms.

What verdict will I receive today?
Will my blood tests show deterioration?
Will the x-rays show suspicious looking spots?
Will I have to fight with the pharmacy for my
pain medications because someone behind
the window thinks I'm just a druggie using AIDS
as an excuse?
Will I have to track the social worker down
because something wasn't right with my paperwork?

And I wonder what other patients think as they watch
from their chairs the steady stream of young men
and occasional young woman who walk through
the door marked exit on their way to the AIDS clinic.

The Tan Plastic Bottle

I look at the small tan plastic bottle
with the wraparound label,
and turn it first to the right,
then to the left.
"Experimental" it says.
I know—I signed those papers.

ddC (dideoxycytidine) a tiny red pill
no bigger than a giant dot,
is only a few micrograms.
It's really not much.
I take one every day.

As magic as this med
is supposed to be, it sets
my nerve endings on fire
making me look like a speckled egg,
with red bumps that line themselves
up in the layers of my skin.

How much do I have to take
before the little tan plastic bottle
delivers its final sentence?
It feels to me like the judge who sits
within the small bottle
has, indeed, made his decision.

II

Going Down
Spring, 1992

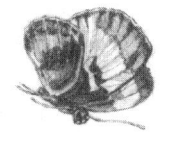

Three AIDS Poems

Two More Weeks

    Two more weeks and I'll be gone.
    Two more weeks and I'll be dead.

Phone calls pour in from Minneapolis-St. Paul,
    New York, Seattle, Portland, Miami, Houston,
        Palm Springs, San Diego,
            England, Israel, and France,
and he tells his friends good-bye. They still call
week after week to see if he's alive.

Neuropathy, and polymyopathy
have settled
    in his feet,
        in his legs,
           in his hips and joints,
until he can no longer walk.
In a monster hospital bed that makes it easier
for us to care for him, he decides to let it go.
No more pills that make his stomach churn.
For what? Six more months of life?
Another year? Maybe two?
No way, he says. Not me, I'll be dead in two more weeks.

And Two More Weeks

A person's body, you'd think, would certainly succumb
confined to bed with no medication for pneumonia,
or food to eat. Only
Roxanol and MS Contin, both morphine meds for pain,
Valium to make the anxiety tolerable,
Acyclovir to keep Herpes from surfacing all over the body,
Fluconazole for that cotton-like yeast called thrush
which would otherwise take over the mouth and throat.
All this he washes down with a cocktail of juice,
    papaya
        mango
            guava and ginger ale.

You'd think that two weeks
was more than adequate for a PWA to die.
For three months, every week
he told his friends good-bye
until one week I said to him—
My son, your body is stronger that we thought.
Your spirit is not ready to take you away.
It could be that you will live beyond the next two weeks
and, God forbid, you should live another month,
or two, or three. I know you are ready to depart,
but only your spirit will know when it's time—

And Weeks and Weeks and Weeks

For three more months he lay and waited with eyes open
watching as the mornings dissolved the blackened night into grey,
and the grey into the light of day. Doves pulled their heads
out from under wings, fluttered about, and then took flight
from a tall pine outside his window.
He talked less and less on the phone with his friends
and those who dropped by stayed only moments.
To all of them he said good-bye and he told them
    I won't be dead, I'll just be gone.

Queer as a Three Dollar Ruble

The three-ruble note
which Jody, my social worker from JFCS,
brought back for me,
a memento from her trip to Russia,
strikes me as queer.

I looked at the strange money,
green and white with a simple pattern
(as three Russians later told me)
of the Kremlin and gerb.

The number three sat in each corner.
It was just the right amount
to buy a bottle of Vodka,
(2.87 rubles to be exact)
which was just enough for three people.

"Jody," I said. "Put this on the wall—by the fairies.
It's as queer as a three dollar ruble.

Trekking with Auntie Ann

We're disabled.
I have AIDS
and Auntie Ann has CFIDS.

We dish long distance almost every day
and hold each other's hand
through the long wires
of hope for cure or relief.

We share doctor horrors,
bouts of night sweats, coughs,
fuzzy thinking, exhaustion and pain
as if we were only on a Nordstrom expedition.

I tell her I'm afraid of the Kabbalah—
the map of consciousness, The Tree of Life—
for fear I'll be swept away by a fast wind
that funnels across the plains.

Auntie Ann wraps herself in white cloth,
breathes into lighted candles,
and chants like a cantor from the bima.
Every day she sits still, like a monk,
and channels prayers into the universe.

I ask what Sadie, the guru Spaniel
is spacing off to today.
More soup bones full of marrow, I'm sure.

Cody Comes to Dish

Cody comes with Marla to dish with me.
His string bean body and high cheek bones
represent the sinewy strength of his heritage—Lakota.
I like Cody, his presence comforts me.

He sports hard-toed, hard-heeled boots,
worn blue jeans with a mean leather belt.
Long light brown hair spindles down
around his neck and street-wise blue eyes.
Doesn't sound much like the person he really is.

"Cody," I say.
"Can I have a braid of your hair?"
"Yes," he says with a laugh.
"I'll use it as a bookmark for my devotional book,
Color of Light."
"All right," Cody says.

Cody draws fairies with wings
who sit on rocks by gentle flowing streams.
Young women's faces framed
with long black braids
and wise old women with long braids turned gray.
Kings of the underground perched on thrones
surrounded by winged guardians.

"Cody," I say. "Place this dainty fairy
to the left of that picture on the wall.
Now down a little.
Over to right.
That's it! That's it! Perfecto!"

Cups of French roast coffee
and Benson & Hedges Ultra Lite cigarettes
we share while we dish about good old Uncle Sam
and Bush's "thousand points of light"
and a society who wants to rub us out.
Now it's time for them to go.
Cody tells me, "Hang in there, Aaron."
"Cody, when you come back, don't forget
that braid of hair."
"I won't," he says.
"And I'll be back for more dish."

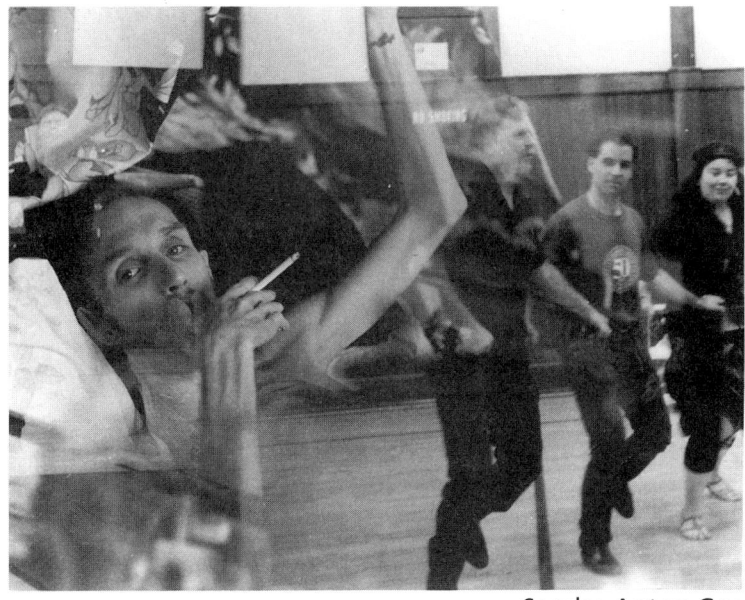

Sandra Anton Gee

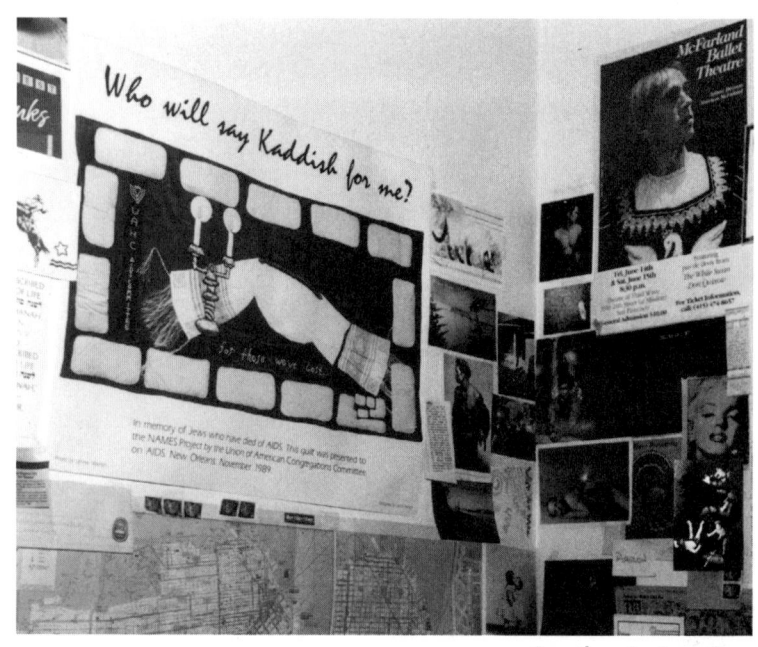

Sandra Anton Gee

Kitchen Walls Talk

Oscar night trips over the Sinai desert
while Madonna hangs, red-framed,
above Lebanon.
A post card of a Madonna momma kitty,
orange striped, stands.
Her two foil cone tits drag the ground
as she watches cockroaches feel their way
across the kitchen walls.
Sandy and Lynn's pencil drawing
of a Madonna cat sports six cone tits.

Leather boys party on the kitchen walls
at the Folsom Street Fair, 1991.
Marilyn puckers up to their bare bottoms
decorated with leather straps and metal rings.
Well-stacked buttocks in tight jeans
stand like a cowboy at attention
with a condom tucked in the back pocket.
The print below says "Safe sex" in Hebrew.

Faster Pussycat bar steps up the pace
and Lipstick Lesbian Julie leaves
her phone number just in case.
Madonna blows kisses to Marilyn.
Totally off the wall, Aaron and Francisco
dressed in nuns' habits, sit on the curb
on Halloween in the Castro.
With glittered-eyes and cornets,
the Sisters of Perpetual Indulgence
with rosaries to their knees, a serious Order,
stand in a circle,
cigarette smoke curling from its center.

Have a heavenly pizza menu at Uncle Vito's,
on the corner of Bush and Powell,
and if you can't make it,
just phone and they'll deliver.
Another party on the wall
and Madonna watches over Chula,
and her children, little Dallas and baby Peter.
Aaron and Marla speak out to teens about
how not to get AIDS.

The kitchen walls reach for the refrigerator door.
Family and friends gather around
and doctor appointments, blood red ribbons,
Chicken Soupers kosher meals schedules,
and AIDS buttons cluster at its bottom.
Marilyn Monroe cradles
Aaron's dead lover, Bob, on the freezer's door.
Spinelli Company magnet sends
Black Hawkers' and Polk Gulchers' for coffee
to drain off the "too much" beer they drink.
A bar ad below says,
"Have a safe sex encounter while you're at it."

Rabbi Stuart plants a "Tree of Life" in Israel
for Aaron and an olive beauty wears
a bikini covered with a hundred
tiny gold and blue Stars of David
London Stuart, nearly blind with CMV,
bungee jumps. And he went all the way
to New Zealand to do it.
Keith frames multiple Marilyns,
by placing them on the diagonal.
They wink at him as he lines
the edges with gold and black.
Cosmos butterflies flit
from get-well cards to Rosh Hashanah cards.
At the top of the page of the kitchen walls,
a poster asks, Who will say Kaddish for me?
It's lost above a map of San Francisco.

Russian / Ukrainian Steps

I walk to the Russian Center, on Sutter and Divisadero,
once a week to take
Russian/Ukrainian character dance lesson
from Leonid Shagalov, Dance Master.

With drobushski steps I mop up my tears.
Fists on hips, chest up (look at those diamonds),
I drop my shoulders and hold my head high.
Leonid shouts turn out, turn out!

> **Yah**, dah dah dah
> **Yah,** dah dah dah
>   **Yah**

Our long dresses sweep patterns
over the dance studio floor.
Blue and red silk scarves flow light
as we move around the room.
In our red shoes we step
softly on the balls of our feet

> **Step**, step step
> **Step**, step step
> **Step**, step step

We form a long line: we hold scarves
corner-to-corner in front of us.
The men burst through the scarves
to take their places.
The music picks up and
I lose my tears in the drobushski steps.

> **Yah**, dah dah dah
> **Yah,** dah dah dah
>   **Yah**

An Unlikely Dessert

It had been a month and a half since Aaron crashed; that is, his body crashed, just completely gave way to the virus that eats up immune cells. The virus sat in the neurological compartments of his brain, waiting to jam signals to the rest of the body. No more walking signals for Aaron; it laid him out flat on his back.

Marla went to see Aaron almost daily and brought hot coffee mocha lattes. She lived on the corner of Van Ness and McAllister, only a few blocks from Aaron. His apartment building, the Rex Arms, was on the corner of Geary and Polk in the Upper Tenderloin, not one of the better areas of San Francisco. But rent was affordable and the neighborhood had its own charm, its own culture. Locals say that Polk Street is the sun belt of the city because the sun breaks through there first while the rest of the city is draped in fog. There is also less wind; only one block west, sharp gusts whip up and down Van Ness.

Marla met Aaron when they were speakers on an AIDS panel. Both had AIDS, and both told how they got AIDS and how not to get it. They spoke to teenagers and college students and anyone who would listen. At that time, she was twenty-seven and he was thirty-one.

Marla walked briskly up Van Ness to Aaron's apartment. He'd nearly died two weeks before, but he was back loud and clear. The wind whipped her almost-dry, dark brown hair around her face. She ducked into a tiny coffee shop and returned to the street with two large Styrofoam cups of steaming coffee mocha lattes.

Aaron's apartment building was red brick and five stories high. The front entrance had wide marble stairs with a black wrought iron gate, Mediterranean style. The street people, Reagan's turned-out, stood on the corner. They didn't match the old architecture of the neighborhood buildings, but there they were, hands out, as they begged for a few cents or just got in the way and tried to look straight into eyes. Marla looked ahead of them as she approached the corner. They grumbled at her as she plowed through them.

She entered the code number on the electronic pad welded onto the gate. The dial tone of each number clicked away, then the telephone rang.

"Hello," a female voice said.

"It's me," said Marla. "I'm here, buzz me in." The door gave a loud growl and unlocked. She pushed the door open and walked up the marble stairs to a larger door with beveled glass and waited again for another lock to release. She pushed the door open with her whole body and stepped inside the old lobby, where the floor was covered with tiny, white hexagonal tiles and a deep red rug that ran from the front door to the elevator. The walls' rich mahogany panels reached almost to the ceiling, and a crystal and brass chandelier branched out from the center of the room.

She entered the old elevator that was lined with brass and mahogany. The elevator rattled as it slowly climbed the inside of the building and took its time to come to a halt at the second floor. She pulled the elevator door and brass gate back just enough to ease through them. As she stepped off, the doors creaked, then closed with a loud snap.

Down the hall to apartment 207 she strode with head held high. Gently, she tapped on the door and then opened it, all the while juggling the two lattes in one hand. As she entered, a thin stream of sandalwood incense curled into the air from an adjustable tray that sat next to Aaron's hospital bed. His mother, Sylvia, was watering the huge spider plants that sat in the kitchen window.

"Hi, Aaron," Marla said. "I got us some mocha lattes." She pulled off a lid and handed the cup to him.

"Ummmm, that tastes soooo good," Aaron said. She stood on her tiptoes and reached over the rails of his bed to give him a kiss. He kissed her and they both giggled softly like two little kids who tell each other secrets.

"You want a cigarette?" Aaron asked her as he picked up the pack of Benson & Hedges Ultra Lites from the bedside tray.

He tapped the pack lightly on the heel of his hand and popped the cigarettes out.

"Yeah," she said.

He handed her a cigarette and then reached toward her as she leaned over the bed. He flicked the lighter and held the flame under the tip of the cigarette.

"Where did you get the lighter?" Marla said. "That is pretty. I want one."

"My mom got it for me," he said. He picked up a small wicker basket with a lid. "See?" He took the lid off and held out a basket filled with what looked like miniature shiny whiskey flasks with black gadgets on one end.

"Oooooh," she said. "Look at all those colors. They're all covered with stars and sparkles."

"Take one."

"You're sure it's O.K.?"

"Yeah, go ahead."

Marla fished around in the small wicker basket and examined each lighter.

"This one is different," she said. "It glitters." Holding it up in the light, she twisted it from side to side. "I like black," she said, squeezing the lighter in her hand.

"Me, too," said Aaron. "It matches our situation, if you know what I mean."

"Yeah, I do." They both giggled.

Marla walked over to a bird cage shaped like a cylinder, with a rounded top. A gray and white rat poked its nose through a pile of rags that lined the bottom of the cage.

"Oh, Barney, is Momma ignoring you?" she said. "You cute little girl." Barney squirmed the top of the pile.

"You want out?" she asked. "Let's go see Dad."

"That's right, you're the mom and I'm the dad," Aaron said. "And my mom is the grandmother." They laughed as Marla opened the cage door. Barney crawled deftly up Marla's arm and sneaked in under her hair to nuzzle her. The rat sniffed all around, then ran to the edge of Marla's shoulder and sat perched like a Greek goddess.

Marla scooped Barney up in her left hand and cradled the lower half of Barney's body with her right hand and raised

Barney up until their noses touched. Barney's little whiskers twitched, and then she licked Marla's nose with her tiny tongue.

"I love you, Barney," Marla told her. She walked toward Aaron's bed as Barney squirmed free onto Marla's shoulder.

"How's your PMS," Aaron asked. "It's about that time again." He lit another cigarette, inhaled, and swallowed his breath before letting it slip back out. "Well, don't forget to put your tampons in the garbage bag. Don't flush them down the toilet. They'll plug it up. You know how this old plumbing is; it can't swallow the tampons without getting stuck."

"I never flush tampons down the toilet," Marla retorted.

Aaron scribbled on a Post-it pad. "Here," he said. "Put this up by the toilet so you girls can see it." Barney peeked out from under Marla's hair as Aaron handed her the note.

Marla looked at Aaron's shaky but forceful handwriting. "DON'T FLUSH TAMPONS DOWN THE TOILET!" she read aloud; then she yelled, "Aaron!" and walked into the bathroom.

Aaron watched from his bed as she placed the note below the toilet paper roll.

"Step aside; let me see," he said. "Over to the right a little. Yeah, that's it. Perfecto."

"Satisfied?"

"Yeah. When is your next doctor's appointment?"

"Next week," she said. "I have to have my T-cell count done again. She paused. "And I need to get my doctor to fill out my SSI/SSD papers. Do you think I'll have any trouble getting my Social Security?"

"What's your last T-cell count?"

"One-hundred-sixty."

"Well, it's below two hundred. You shouldn't have any problem, but you never know," Aaron said. "It just depends on who you get at the front desk. They're so fucked up they don't know what they're doing most of the time, and most of them don't give a damn about PWA's. At least that's my experience." He took another drag from his cigarette. "It's a socially unacceptable disease, you know."

"Yeah, I know," Marla said. "Some of them can sure make you feel like shit. *You look just fine. Why can't you work? You don't look sick. Go get a job.*"

"Yeah, well, let them try AIDS and see how quick they show up at the Social Security window!" Aaron said. Marla reached for Barney and scratched behind her ears.

"You want me to read from your *Color of Light* book?" she asked.

"Yeah, sounds like a good idea. What day is it?"

"It's May fifth."

"You know, I know Perry Tilleraas. He wrote that," said Aaron. "He gave me my first copy. Go ahead, read."

Marla thumbed through the pages and read the meditation.

"I really like that," said Aaron.

"Yeah, I have to remind myself to think about the moment I'm in," Marla added. "It's hard not to think about the fact that I probably won't live a full life. No, change that to a *long* life."

For a split second Marla visualized how it was when her late best girlfriend she had met in an AIDS support group went through what Aaron was going through now. The two young women used to talk about how surprised they were to discover they had AIDS when they didn't even use IV drugs. It was just sex, straight sex.

"Just remember, Marla, take good care of yourself. Keep one foot on your doctors' necks, and make them tell you the truth. Don't let them kiss you off. Keep up with the information." Aaron waved his hand around above his head. "It's the living in the moment that counts. That's what gets you through. It makes you see life differently."

"You're so strong, Aaron. I could never be strong like you or put up with the pain you do." Barney ran down Marla's arm into her lap and circled about, then up to the back of her neck.

"You'll get stronger. You're already stronger."

"I wonder what will happen to Barney if I die before she does," Marla said. "I don't know who'll take her."

"How old is Barney?"

"She's three years old."

"You know, rats have a life span of about three to four years. She could die before you do."

"I hadn't thought about that."

"If Barney dies before you do, you have to bury her on top of her dad," Aaron said. "Give her a Jewish burial."

"And wrap her up in white cloth," she said. Both of them giggled while Barney continued to roam around on Marla's shoulders.

"And don't forget to put her little tallis around her neck and cover her head with a tiny yarmulke."

"Your mom can make the yarmulke."

"Can you imagine what the Rabbi would say? A kosher rat with a traditional Jewish burial." They burst into laughter as Barney poked her head out from under Marla's hair and looked around.

"Aaron," Marla asked, "How am I going to get Barney to Portland?"

Aaron thought for a minute and then yelled to his mom, just like old times, "Mom, how do we get Barney to Portland from San Francisco if she's dead? Wouldn't she rot in the mail?" Aaron's mom peeked around the corner of the kitchen door.

"Several years ago I mailed your grandparents a special cake that I had to pack in dry ice and ship air freight. Today you could Federal Express her on dry ice. Just wrap her up good, put her in a solid box, and send her off. If they ask what's in the box, tell them it's a perishable special dessert that needs to be delivered immediately."

"Perfect! Perfecto!" Aaron said. " Where do you get dry ice?"

"Any ice cream store, like a Baskin Robbins."

"Now we have to have someone make sure Barney is buried on top of me, *traditionally*."

"But who's going to do that?" Marla asked.

Aaron and Marla looked at each other and chimed, "MOM!"

Aaron's mom's eyes widened. They burst into laughter as Barney raced out to the edge of Marla's shoulder, panned the room, and sniffed while her whiskers twitched.

Snap Trap

My son and I were trapped for four months,
    prisoners behind bars,
        in his Rex Arms apartment.

AIDS snapped the trap
    tight over Aaron's legs
        so he couldn't walk.

While he lay in a hospital bed
    the virus curled
        his strong bones.

His butterfly shoulders
    which swam so hard, wilted
        like a cut rose without water.

For six months
    he rarely flinched
        as he stared at his death.

His last day of life, the trap snapped open,
    he woke up, and
        conducted his final exit.

Breathing: An Unrealized Meditation

April 1992: My new sleeping quarters are my son's single futon in his studio apartment, barely large enough to house his monstrous bed. Only two steps away I listen for each breath as if he were a new newborn.

> It's familiar—the helplessness,
> the full dependence on me.
>
> When he was growing up, I would slip into the room
> he shared with his little brother and lean over
> to watch them breathe.
> I'd listen to their dream noises
> and wonder what they saw.

Sixteen, he got past me to a kegger. His swim team friends deposited him at our front gate, blue with alcohol. I watched him all night counting each breath. He let me into the bathroom where he sat on the toilet, head in his hands, and said, "If this is what it takes to be a man, they can forget it."

August 1992: My son has moved
to Coming Home Hospice. My bed covers
one tiny corner in a room just big enough for a nun—
three quilts layered on the floor. Now four steps
from his bed where he lies, I watch him breathe.
Waiting for his last breath.

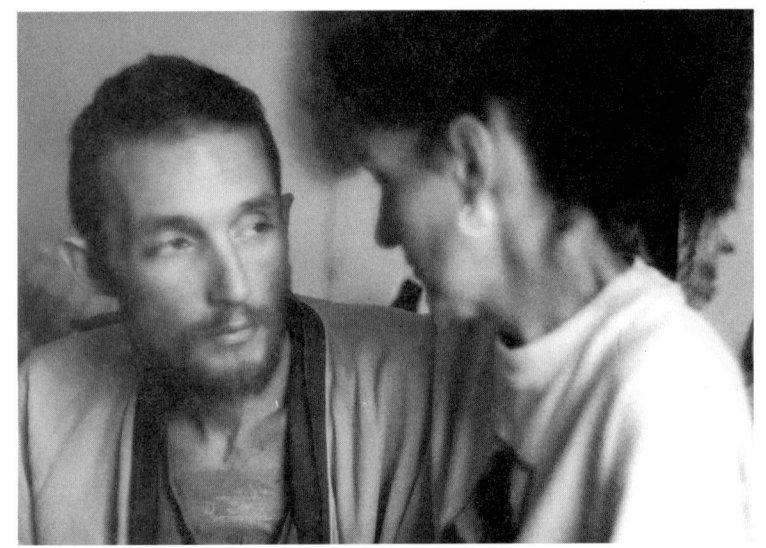

Sandra Anton Gee

Waking Up to Die

Skin lies draped over his bony body.
All day the sockets sit deep with sleep
like screws set into drilled holes
in a 4 by 4 post. I sit and wait.
I send for the nurse to check him.

I think it's close to time. The nurse
lifts his lids and assures me it's not time,
he's just sleeping, soundly.
But I'm not so sure. I sit and wait
all day and all night.

Next morning sleep lifts the lids of the sockets.
Confused, he shows us his carefully guarded valium. He has
stashed twelve pale yellow pills
because he thought the doctor might discontinue it. He says I
need my valium where I'm going.

At forty minutes past high noon,
October 10, 1992,
our sleeper wakes up to die.
He directs each person
about what to do next
and tells us I love you all–Shalom.

Rainbow Butterfly

"Aaron Aaron, tomorrow is the day that Moses died,"
Rabbi Weiss said to me.

    Is it time? Is it time?

Today tomorrow is here.
I look at the walls of soft pink
covered with pictures, posters, cards,
and feather boas that look like red mink.

This is my room, I know why I'm here.

The warm morning sun beams through
illuminating pots and vases of flowers.
Lines of light fan out to touch
the end of my bed.

Leo, Leo, my breath is going.
Today I spread my wings.
This is really hard work

Johna, Johna, comfort me.
Mom may not make it in time.

Mary, Mary, sit with me.
You can keep me company.

Sandy, Sandy, is that you?
I reach out to touch her hand.

Mom, Mom, you're here, you're here!
She climbs in bed with me.

Jim, Jim, there you are.
Behind my mom you stand.

Irving, Irving, standing by the door
to share in my final event.

Janet, Janet, can I have more?
Cocktail time it is.

My eyes, my eyes, I cannot see.
Everyone grab an arm and a leg.
I want to be touched.

The oxygen line, I hand it back.

My mom begins to talk. "Aaron, do you remember Valentine
waits under a big oak tree for Richard?
Your Bob is there, too. Wait under that tree
and some day Richard and I will join you there.

Aaron, I see you burst out of your cocoon,
a butterfly to be. And there you are flying over
the rainbow with your butterfly wings. Now
you're coming back under the rainbow.
With gentle poise and magnificence,
you turn and glide into the rainbow.
Each color touches the tips of your butterfly wings."

"Puppy, Puppy," Janet says to me. "Open up, open up."

    It is time. It is time.

With my right hand in Sandy's hands,
and my left hand in Mom's hands,
as the lighted candle's bursting brightness
fills my room, I look at it as best I can
and begin to take that final step.

But before I do, I want you to know:
    I love you all—Shalom.

Metamorphosis

The telephone rings.
Oh, God, the day has arrived.
It catches me as I bathe
as if getting ready for a renewal,
a rebirth.

Why, why, and then again,
why not me?
Am I so privileged
that I should be passed over?
No, but let me trade places,
it would make more sense.

Run! Run!
I catch the elevator.
Hurry! Hurry!
Not a minute to be wasted.
It might be over before I get there.
Slowly, the elevator drops,
drops, drops, eleven stories.

Oh, God—no taxis.
Not one in sight.
A small flower shop,
all colors of the rainbow
stare me in the face.
    May I use your phone? It's an emergency.
I wait and pace
back and forth
on the sunlit sidewalk.
Call again.
    "Sorry lady, we'll be there as soon as we can."
Suddenly a beat up old taxi
comes down the street.
Run! Run!
    Taxi! Taxi! It's an emergency!

He drives too slow.
I direct him,
tears stream down my face.
All this traffic
where did it come from?
And on a Saturday morning,
the day that Moses died.
Hurry! Get me there in time.

Finally he decides to accommodate me,
weaves in and out between the cars.
Now we are at Eighteenth and Diamond streets,
San Francisco.
So much traffic no turn can be made.
I burst out the cab door,
with one foot high in the air
and hand the driver a twenty dollar bill.
   "Hey, lady. Wait. Here's your change."

I run down Diamond Street
to a soft rose-colored
two-story stucco building.
Billie sits on the steps,
he lives here now.
He looks at me.
"I'm sorry, Sylvia."
I pat him on the back
and know that he will be next.

Can I go in?
Into the tiny pink room
just big enough for a nun,
holy as it seems, I rip off my sandals.
I shake at the sight of my first born.
I am so scared.
Just like I was thirty-one-and-a-half years ago.

I leap over the bottom of the bed
and land next to his left side.

He moves a little in his upright position,
oxygen line hooked up.
I could kill him by moving around on his bed,
it wouldn't take much.
He looks at me and whispers,
> *I'm sorry, Mom.*

I cry and try to be brave
only to see that he
is really the brave one.
> It's not O.K. that you should die.
> But since you are, I'll stay with you.

He breathes fast and heavy now.
There is that rattle in the throat.
With eyes wide open
he directs the nurse, asks for pain relief.
She checks with Dr. Swift and obliges.

He sees the end,
lifts off the oxygen line
and hands it to the nurse.

I look left to the wall,
there's a picture of him with his lover, Bob,
all curled up together smiling.
And next to them, a picture
of where he'll rest.
He's prepared for this event.
I'm resigned.

I walk him over and through the rainbow
as he breaks out of his safe cocoon
Rabbi Weiss helped him build.
Momentum gathers
as he spreads his butterfly wings.
He utters his last words with his last breath,
> *I love you all. Shalom.*

I hang over his body.
And weep and hold his hand in mine.

The room glows
and I feel every inch packed tight
with molecules that rush up the walls
and line the corners and the ceiling.
It's full, soothing, sad.
Magnificent.

My baby gone.
I've just given birth
to him again.
Only this time
I don't get to keep him.
Except—deep within.

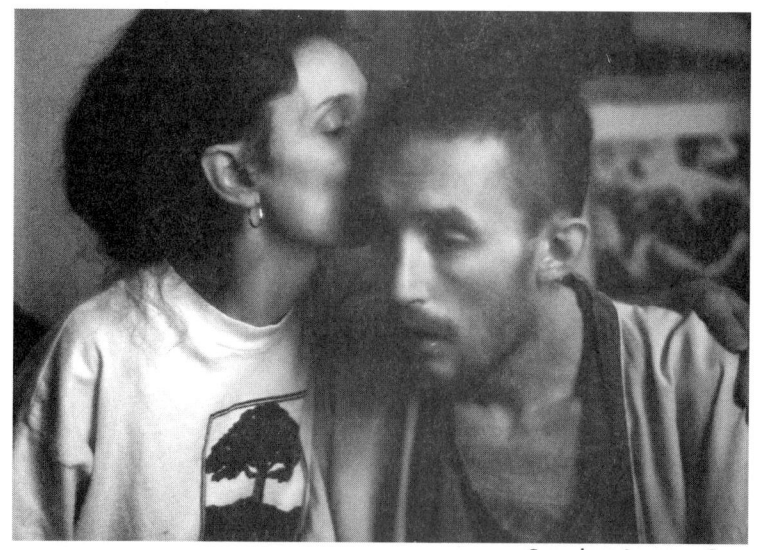

Sandra Anton Gee

III

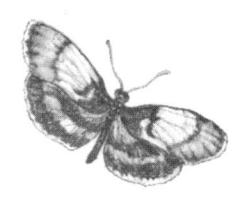

Universal Traveler
October 10, 1992

Fearful Hierarchies

When I came back to Portland,
after my son had died,
the Oregon Citizens Alliance
was in full tilt with their campaign
against gays and lesbians.
My anger burned as they vomited
like volcanoes from the ring of fire.
"Look at all the trash in the libraries:
Walt Whitman's *Leaves of Grass*
Emily Dickinson's poems
Gertrude Stein's *Autobiography of Alice B. Toklas*
Tennessee Williams' *Streetcar Named Desire*
And you don't want one for a neighbor.
It might rub off on you."

The OCA tried to convince everyone.
Even Blacks and Jews they tried to enlist,
saying "The Bible says."
These pillowed-cased knights hate anyone
different.

I wanted to shake the Lon Mabons and say,
"Wake up foolish ones, look around,
check the facts.
Talk with gay and lesbian and bisexual people.
You, too, are sexual with a history.
You must have forgotten
how it was when you were sixteen,
driven by the testosterone
lined thick in your veins."

The fear-driven ballot measure cut
deep into my core with its family values.
Which meant, "Off with your heads,
you heathen ones, let's burn you at the stake."

No Clue

YOU!
    YOU!
        YOU!
        You don't have a clue.
        You have *not* walked in my shoes.
        Been where I've been.
        Seen what I've seen.
        Felt what I have felt.
        Know what I know.

        No, you really don't have a clue.
        How could you?
        You weren't there.
        How would you know what it was like to watch
        your child dissolve before your eyes?

        And how can any sane person pass judgment
        on another for self-expression, or for whom they love?
        Do you know that nature stands in the doorway
        of life and waits for opportune times to step in
        to express itself at the expense of one of us?

        Any one of us can get AIDS;
        we're not immune
        just because of how we are sexually
        or who we have sex with,
        or that we have it the correct way.
        What delusions we place ourselves in.

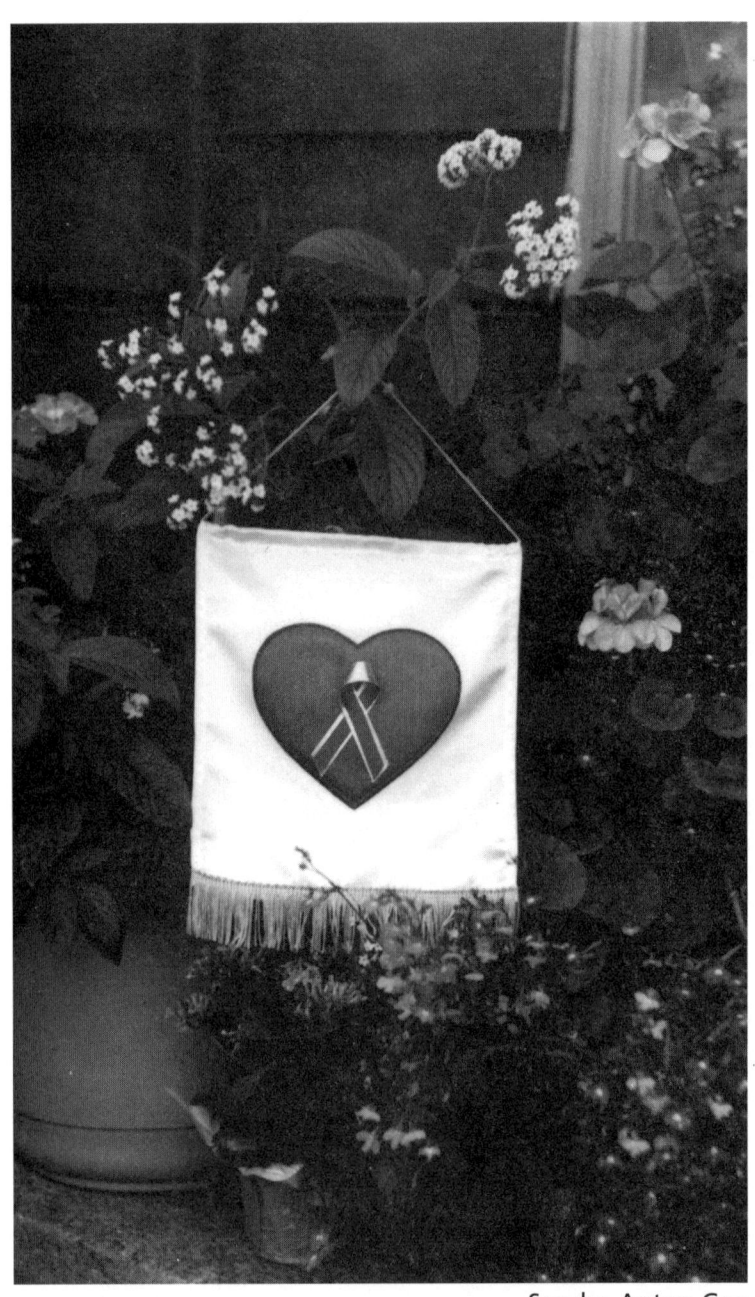

Sandra Anton Gee

A Different Kind of Veteran

My MOMS purple heart hangs
in the window by the front door.
It's slashed with a red ribbon.
Yellow-orange leaves with blood red
cover the front porch—
my son's favorite time of year.

After he died, I returned to work.
I wanted a bereavement group:
Cascade AIDS Project Wednesday evenings.
I asked for four swing shift Wednesdays off.
I offered to work weekends.

But the supervisor told me,
The work group has had enough of you.
Someone suggested I start my own group.
You're so good at the dying stuff.
Some coworkers' words singed my mind.
I'm sorry your son died even though he sinned.
My carpool friend said, *You're like a Vietnam vet.*
You've come home and nobody knows where you've been.

Driving Home

The leaves fall
and overlay one another.
Winds begin and with them the rain,
then ice and snow.

It's midnight,
my work finished.
I drive home cautiously
up the steep hill with

cemeteries on either side.
I wonder, is he cold? My son.
I want to go home
and get electric blankets,
        heavy blankets,
              aluminum blankets

and take them back to where he lies
on top of the hill
where he watches
over Portland.

I want to cover him up,
wrap him up,
so that he is warm.
It is not right
that he should remain cold.

I want to warm him up,
bring him back to life
so he can finish living,
finish being who he is.
Then he could tell about AIDS.

אהבת שלום

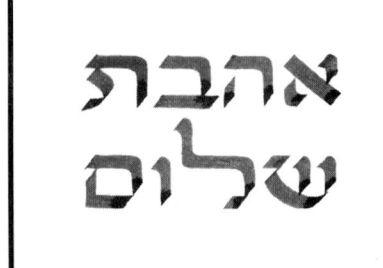

Judy Horowitz

Love of Peace
(Ahavai Sholom)

Eleven months later
the pain sits in my heart.
Will it ever go away?
Will I ever think straight again
or is this forever?
But I don't want to loose the pain.

It's time to unveil the stone.
Fine lines surround his name,
his birth date,
his death date,
with the Star of David in the middle.
His last words—
> *I love you all, Shalom—*
sit at the bottom of the gray granite.

Bunched up starlings scream
and I hear his words—
> *Mom, just because I die doesn't mean you have to—*
I stand above the gray granite
and read to my son a poem
about the last few hours of his rainbow life.

Rabbi Shoenberg and family and friends
surround his grave
to chant the Kaddish.
The starlings' scream crescendos,
then drops off into total silence.

All too soon we leave
the quiet green lawns
dotted with granite markers
protected by firs, cedars,
and old maples.

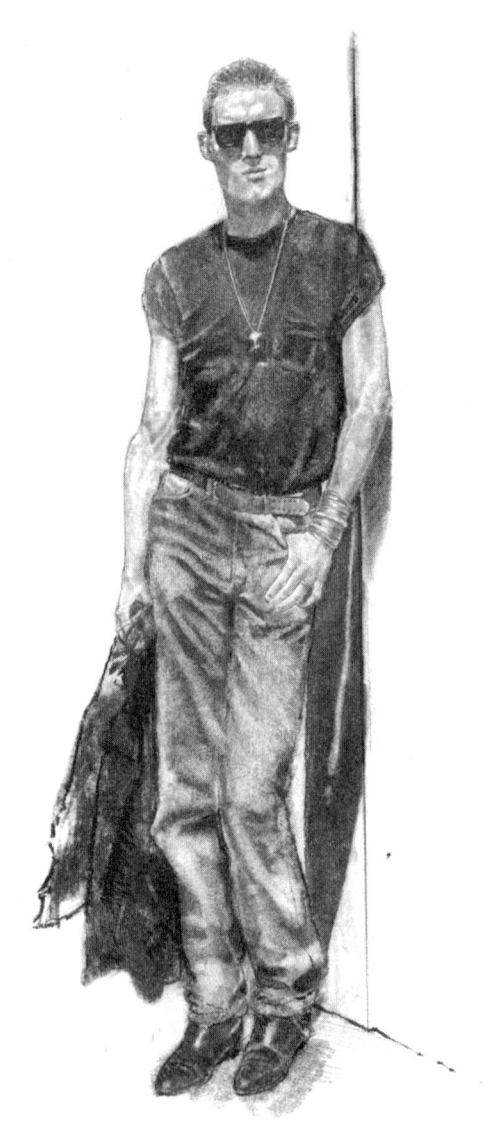

A Gala Event for Sandy Kovtun
Recognized for outstanding volunteer service
March 25, 1995, Weston St. Francis, San Francisco

I didn't make it to Aaron's grave
before I left for San Francisco
to say good-bye again.
I wanted to tell him
that Sandy's being honored
at a dinner and dance.
I knew he loved to talk about her looks,
how beautiful she is all dressed up.
Just like he did when she dropped by his apartment
on her way to a wedding.

He'd tell her, "Let me look at you."
And then he'd smile.
"Turn around. Gorgeous! Gorgeous!
Now let me see your jewelry.
Nice. Nice. Tell Merle to buy you more.
Yes, yes, we're going to Paris.
Put you on the runway.
We'll knock 'em dead,
make lots of money."
All this he'd say in one breath
and then he'd laugh.

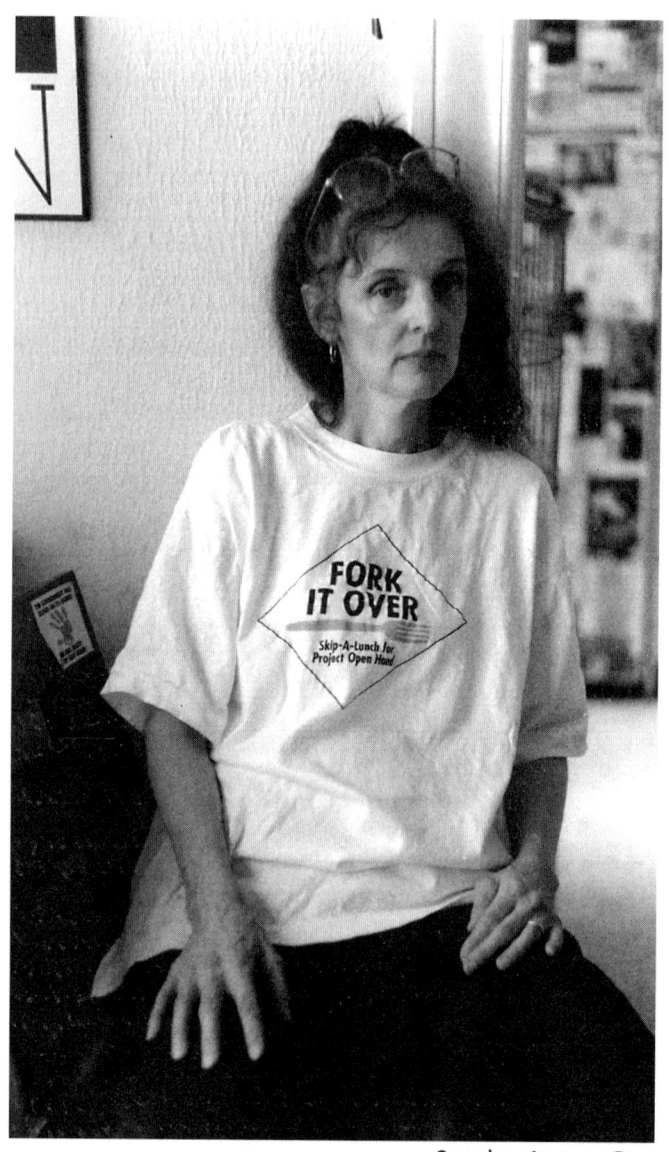

Sandra Anton Gee

I Sat on Tears

When you were infected
    no one knew
        of HIV.

I didn't want to injure
    you any more because
        you couldn't reverse the HIV.

You worried about the pain
    you threw my way,
        so I sat on my tears.

I was afraid
    that once they started
        they'd never stop.

The HIV,
    the tears
        are not your fault.

I sat so hard on those tears, now
    all I can muster is a shallow pool
        of salt.

Marlboro Spurs
(This statement about the Marlboro Cigarette Company was taken from a conversation with my son.)

Today's mail brought a birthday present for my dead son, addressed to him in wedding style print from the Marlboro Cigarette Company. Marlboro sent cards the last two years. Last year I wrote on one of those cards. I told them my son was dead and sent it back. It felt like some mean trick had been played intentionally. As I tore open the wrapping, the gift began to tear my heart into shreds.

My son told me before he died that he'd quit smoking Marlboros because Marlboro had supported anti-gay and -lesbian legislation. So the gay community boycotted Marlboro and ever since, my son has received a birthday card. But this year, he received a T-shirt—blue-gray and navy-blue, with a pocket over the heart for his pack of cigarettes.

Doesn't Marlboro know that people are dying of AIDS too? Especially gay people? Is this an act of remembrance or is it an act of meanness? Has their boycott led Marlboro to court the gay community with well-made T-shirts? Have they felt the loss of dollars?

Even the large red envelope said happy birthday in giant black letters. And wouldn't you know, the card showed a beautiful scene of the northern plains, maybe in Wyoming, complete with red rim rocks, a green prairie freshened by a recent rain, and a half dozen or so good-looking cowboys on sorrel horses, and not one rainbow, but two.

On the back of the extra large T-shirt, from shoulder to shoulder, three pairs of legs, boots with spurs in place, stand at cowboy attention on top of the Marlboro emblem, encircling the words MARLBORO COUNTRY STORE with a big M in the center.

Is this gift to the dead son a gift of remembrance or is it a gift of meanness? The mother of the son wants to know.

Large Pink Duofold

At thirty-five degrees that damp
Portland air seeps through the pores
of my thin layer of skin—no fat
cushions the cold air.

This calls for Duofold thermal underwear.
Outer layer, fifty-five percent polyester
and forty-five percent wool. Inner layer,
one-hundred percent Thermax polyester.

I pull the pink underwear bottoms
(women's large size) over my sock-padded foot,
and drop the pink underwear top
over my head. The pink hangs on me
like cloth draped over old chairs.

I cinch the waist with a stretchy belt.
I bought them for my son's frail body.
It feels strange to wear his clothes,
and yet there is a comfort
in knowing that these touched his skin—
the life I gave him now gone.

April 9, 1996

On Aaron's birthday
I pulled grass, loosened dirt,
planted columbines,
in remembrance.

I wanted to chase the moles
down the runways they'd woven
through the mind of my yard.
Instead, I did what I knew Aaron would've done.

I cleared paths from curb to walkway
to fill them with pea-sized gravel and concrete pavers.
I turned the compost of vegetables gone bad.
I planted peas in a straight line in full sun.

After a day in the backyard
of my mind—just like Aaron,
I fluffed around in the kitchen,
drank a cup of French roast,
and smoked a Winston Ultra Lite,
only my cigarette sat invisible between my fingers.

Edward Scissorhands **Bouquet**

Christmas night, 1996, my roommate, Kim, and I
watched the video *Edward Scissorhands*.
Edward crept about an Addam's Family house.
He hid as if in a closet with doors locked
and no air to breathe.

I thought about Aaron and the closet door he kicked open,
the fresh air he sucked in. I remember his laugh
when he and his friends
talked about Edward Scissorhands snipping away.

I had an old bouquet of dried flowers I brought back
from San Francisco. Aaron had arranged them
while he lay in bed wasting away.
Faded yellow, purple, rose, and blue strawflowers
poked their heads through the dried baby's breath branches,
sticky with gray snow dust.

I cut the bouquet into tiny pieces
just as Edward Scissorhands
sculpted the neighborhood's dogs and green bushes,
and even the women's hair.
Like Aaron, Edward snipped his way back to his beginnings,
and I laid the Scissorhands' trimmings on Aaron's grave.

Throwing Out Tea Bags

Friday
evening
the full moon
tugged
on the insides
of me
like it pulls
the waves
of large bodies
of water.
I fished
through a drawer
full of
all kinds of teas.
Boxes
big enough
to hold
twenty
tea bags.
Small
cylindrical cans
of loose tea.
Plastic bags
filled
with loose tea
and tea bags.

Teas
from a previous marriage
gone stagnate.
Teas from my dead son's
apartment
I'd cleaned out
four years ago.
And teas I bought
for my Russian friends
when I first moved
into this house.
I stood
in the center
of my small kitchen
and looked
at the garbage can.
I lifted the lid
and laid
the stale tea bags
steeped in memories
into it and shut the lid.

      English Breakfast (generic)
Gypsy Cold Care
    Good Earth (original)
        Pompadour's Hibiscus
    Sunrise Orange Mint
Raspberry Lemon Grass
    Rose Hips
       Comfrey
         Chamomile
           Licorice

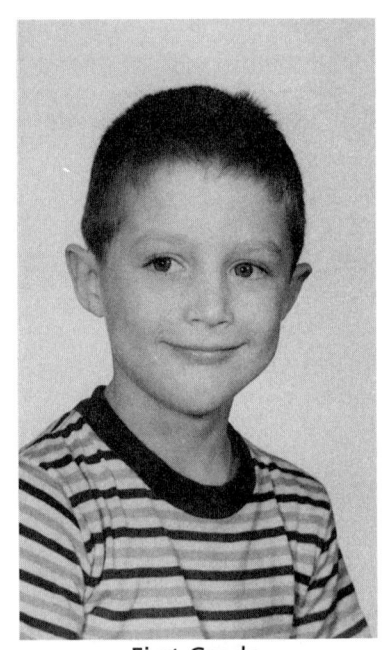

First Grade

Molecular Journeys

We've always been
We are
We always will be
> Something

We are molecules
Bound together
By the dance of life

We may not understand
All that we are
But we definitely are
> Something

Even after our death
Trees reach into the ground
And pull us back to life

Urns in niches wait
For dispersal of their living sand
When the walls collapse

We've always been
We are
We always will be
> Something

Glossary

AIDS acquired immunodeficiency syndrome.

ARC AIDS Related Complex.

Bima a platform in the front of the room in a synagogue.

CDC Center for Disease Control.

CFIDS Chronic Viral Fatigue Syndrome.

Color of Light AIDS daily devotional book by Perry Tilleraas, who died from AIDS in the early 1990's.

Dementia Alzheimer's-like condition some PWA's develop in the later stages of AIDS.

ddC (dideoxycytidine) antiviral drug.

Dish to gossip.

Ferric form of iron.

Gerb Russian seal used on rubles (paper monetary notes).

Hematite form of iron.

Herpes sexually transmitted disease or shingles.

HIV Positive person who tests positive for the retrovirus that causes AIDS.

JFCS Jewish Family *and* Children's Services.

Kaddish mourner's prayer, an ancient Aramaic poem recited during synagogue and burials.

Kaposi's sarcoma slow progressive cancer characterized by the development of bluish-red cutaneous nodules.

Kipa Hebrew. The skullcap worn by Jews. In Yiddish, yarmulke.

Mohs scale scale of hardness for minerals.

MOMS Mothers Organizing MotherS,
66 Cleary Court, Suite #2
San Francisco, California 94109
Phone or Fax (415) 673-8350

Neuropathy abnormal and unusual degenerative state of the nervous system or nerves.

OCA Oregon Citizen's Alliance.

O.I. opportunistic infection.

Perfecto absolutely perfect.

Pneumocystis carenii microorganism (bacteria) that usually infects the lungs of a immune compromised person.

PWA person with AIDS.

Scared of That term used by the gay community to acknowledge a person's moxie. Book title.

Shabbas candles special candle lighted at sundown every Friday, usually eighteen minutes before sunset and approximately forty minutes before nightfall.

Shingles folk term for the virus Herpes zoster.

STD sexual transmitted disease.

Tallis, talit, tallith rectangular prayershawl made out of either wool or silk with either blue or black stripe at both ends.

Thrush disease that is caused by a fungus (Candida Albicans) occurring especially in infants and children and marked by white patches in the mouth. PWA's are very susceptible to thrush.

VNH Visiting Nurses Hospice of San Francisco.

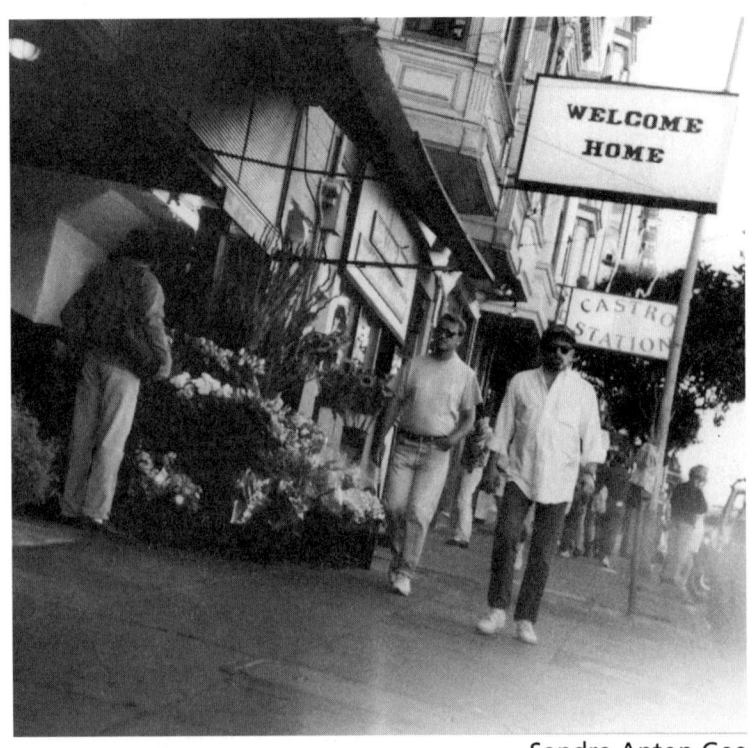

Sandra Anton Gee

Please continue to donate to the AIDS organizations of your choice.